MW00713888

Keto Cocktails

2 Books in 1: Create your Favorite Ketogenic Friendly Alcohol Drinks at Home to Lose Weight and Have Fun with your Friends

Jenny Kern

Keto Cocktails for Beginners

Create your Favorite Keto Friendly Alcohol Drinks at Home to Lose Weight and Have Fun with your Friends

Jenny Kern

Table Of Contents

Introduction

Are you eager to know how to make perfect keto cocktails for your family, friends or guests? What ingredients to put in sangria? Which method to choose to prepare Daiquiri? Which alcohol base is best for Mojito? What drinks serve as excellent aperitifs or digestives? This cookbook for both professional bartenders and home cocktail aficionados answers all of the above questions and more. I hope that the cocktails I have to offer you can have fun in their realization and that you will like it. Enjoy.

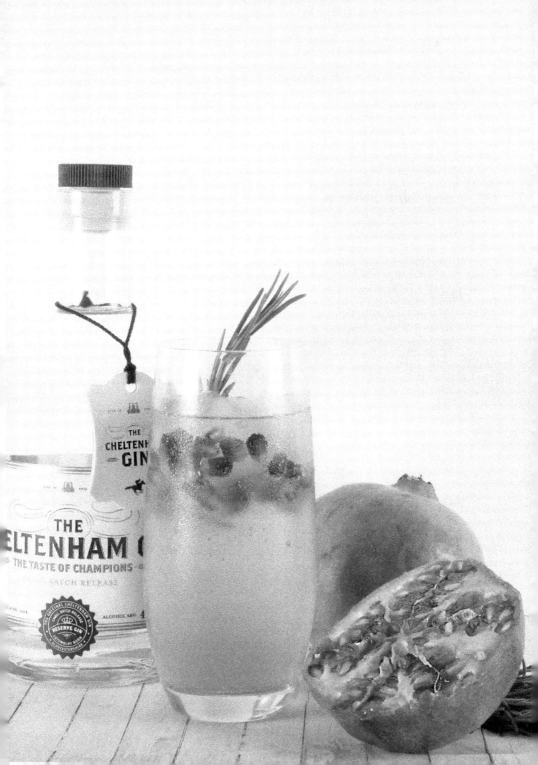

Wine and Champagne Keto Cocktails

Mimosa cocktail

Preparation time: 10 minutes

Servings: 2

Ingredients:

5 teaspoons or 1/2 b

Rut sparkling wine

5 teaspoons or 1/2 orange juice

1slice of orange to garnish

Directions:

To prepare the Mimosa, squeeze the orange - about half - and pour the juice into a flute.

Add the very cold brut sparkling wine

From the remaining orange, make a crescent-shaped slice, slightly cutting the slice so that you can apply it to the glass.

Your Mimosa cocktail is ready to be sipped.

Tips:

Mimosa cocktails should be consumed immediately.

Passion mimosa

Preparation time: 10 minutes

Servings: 2

Ingredients:

4 tablespoons of passion fruit juice

1 tablespoon of triple sec

5oz. of champagne

Strawberry to decorate

Directions:

Pour the passion fruit juice into a champagne flute.

Also, add the triple sec and finally the champagne.

With the bar spoon, mix gently, preventing the release of the bubbles from champagne.

Wash and cut the strawberries in half and use them to decorate the glass.

Alternatively, you can use mimosa sprigs to be fixed on the fluted stem.

Champagne Margaritas

Preparation time: 5 minutes

Servings: 2

Ingredients:

1 bottle champagne

½ cup orange liqueur

1 cup tequila

½ cup fresh lime juice

2 ounces simple syrup

¼ cup fresh mint leaves

Salt, for rim

Lime wedge, for rim

Directions:

Run the lime wedge around the rim of each glass and dip in the salt.

Combine champagne, orange liqueur, tequila, lime juice, mint, and simple syrup in a large pitcher. Mix well.

Pour into glasses and garnish with a lime wedge.

Sicilian Sunset Champagne with Lemon

Preparation time: 10 minutes

Servings: 4

Ingredients:

1 cup Prosecco, which is an Italian sparkling wine

2 cups ice cubes

1 cup cranberry juice

Zest from 2 lemons

1 cup orange juice

Directions:

Add the ice cubes to a pitcher.

Pour the Prosecco wine into the pitcher, along with cranberry and orange juice. Stir the mixture well.

Get champagne flutes. Pour the mixture into them.

Sprinkle with lemon zest, and serve.

Pomegranate Champagne

Preparation time: 10 minutes

Servings: 6

Ingredients:

1 750-ml bottle sparkling wine or champagne

¼ cup brandy

½ cup ginger ale

4 cups ice, crushed

2 cups pomegranate juice

Optional ingredient: pomegranate seeds

Directions:

Mix the wine, brandy, ginger ale, ice, and pomegranate juice in a pitcher.

Pour the mixture into glasses.

Garnish each glass with pomegranate seeds, if using.

Amaretto Cherry Cocktail

Preparation time: 10 minutes

Servings: 2

Ingredients:

1 cup champagne

1 cup fresh cherries, pitted

2 cups brut prosecco, chilled

½ cup egg whites, pasteurized

½ cup lemon juice

Directions:

Add the cherries to a glass jar. Pour the amaretto over the cherries in the container, and cover. Gently shake before storing for around 48 hours to two weeks in a dry and cool place.

After storing it for a certain period, use a sieve to strain the cherries into a bowl. Reserve the cherries and amaretto since you will be using them later.

Pour the amaretto in a quart-sized mason jar or a cocktail shaker. Mix in the egg whites and lemon juice. Add ice to the mixture.

Cover the jar or shaker and shake it for around fifteen seconds.

Strain the mixture in champagne flutes or chilled cocktail coupes. Each flute or coupe should have around one-fourth cup of the mixture.

Top the drink with one-fourth cup prosecco. Use the cherries soaked in amaretto as garnishing.

Serve this drink right away.

Party Mimosa

Preparation time: 10 minutes

Servings: 12

Ingredients:

1 12-oz. can mango-apricot nectar

3/4 c. cold water

1 12-oz. can pineapple juice

1 750-ml. bottle cold champagne

1 6-oz. can undiluted orange juice concentrate, frozen then thawed

Directions:

Stir the pineapple juice, orange juice concentrate, water, and apricot nectar in a pitcher. Make sure to mix everything well.

Pour the sparkling wine into the mixture. Serve.

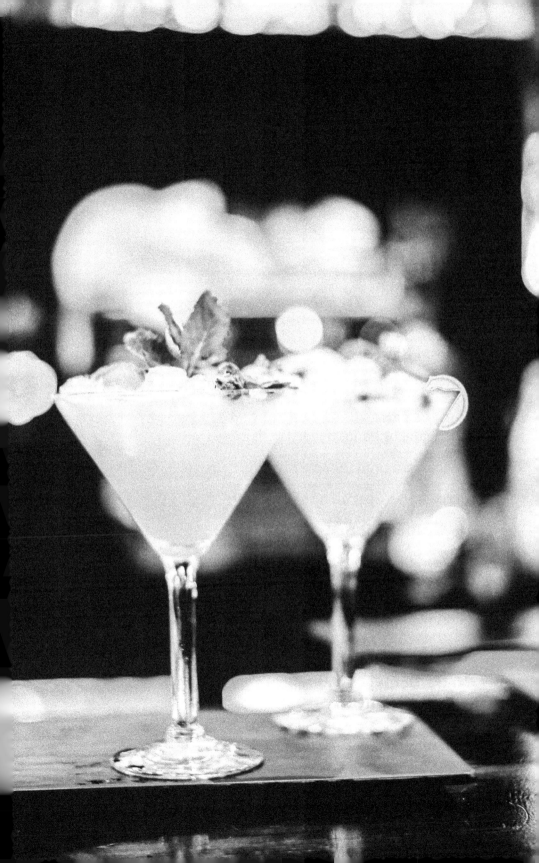

Gin Keto Cocktails

Martini Royale cocktail

Preparation time: 5 minutes

Servings: 1

Ingredients:

Pink Martini

An orange wedge

Martini Prosecco Sigillo Blu

Directions:

Put 1/2 part of Pink Martini and 1/2 part of Prosecco in a hurricane or balloon glass with lots of ice.

Squeeze an orange wedge inside.

Serve for an aperitif or after dinner.

Grapefruit Sangria

Preparation time: 10 minutes

Servings: 7

Ingredients:

½ cup gin or vodka, whichever you prefer

½ cup ruby red grapefruit, cut into four equivalent portions, then cut

½ cup Simple Syrup

½ cup white grapefruit, cut into half-wheels

1 bottle pinot grigio

soda water, as required

Directions:

Mix all of the ingredients apart from the soda water in a big ceramic or glass container.

Place in your fridge, covered, for a minimum of 4 hours (preferably overnight).

Serve over ice and top with soda water.

French 75

Preparation time: 10 minutes

Servings: 2

Ingredients:

8 milliliters sugar syrup

15 milliliters lemon juice

45 milliliters London dry gin

top with champagne brut

Directions:

Shake the first three ingredients with ice and strain into chilled glass. Top with champagne. Garnish using lemon zest twist.

Fog Chopper

Preparation time: 10 minutes

Servings: 2

Ingredients:

15 milliliters almond (orgeat) syrup

15 milliliters amontillado sherry

15 milliliters lemon juice

15 milliliters London dry gin

22 milliliters Cognac V.S.O.P.

45 milliliters light white rum

45 milliliters orange juice

Directions:

Shake the first six ingredients with ice and strain into ice-filled glass. Float sherry on top of the drink. Garnish using an orange wedge.

Flash Tornado

Preparation time: 10 minutes

Servings: 2

Ingredients:

30 milliliters dry vermouth

30 milliliters London dry gin

30 milliliters orange juice

3 dashes peach bitters

Directions:

Shake ingredients with ice and strain into chilled glass. Garnish using orange zest twist.

Enigma Martini

Preparation time: 10 minutes

Servings: 2

Ingredients:

15 milliliters apricot brandy liqueur

15 milliliters lime juice

30 milliliters dry vermouth

60 milliliters London dry gin

Directions:

Shake ingredients with ice and strain into chilled glass. Garnish using lime zest twist.

English Martini

Preparation time: 10 minutes

Servings: 2

Ingredients:

30 milliliters elderflower liqueur

1 sprig rosemary

75 milliliters London dry gin

Directions:

Strip rosemary leaves from stem and muddle in the base of the shaker. Put in the other ingredients, shake with ice, and strain into chilled glass.

Garnish using rosemary sprig.

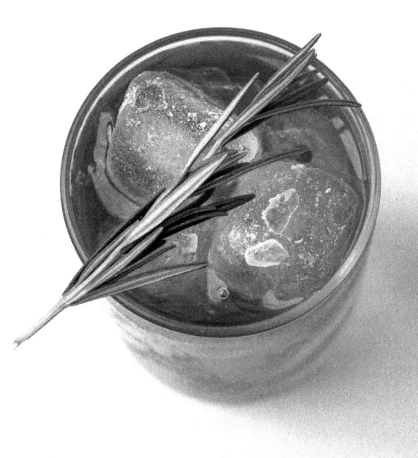

Whiskey Keto Cocktails

Tennessee Rye Brunswick cocktail

Preparation time: 10 minutes

Servings: 2

Ingredients:

2 parts of Jack Daniele's Tennessee rye

¾ claret red wine

½ simple syrup

¾ lemon juice

Orange slice

Cherry

Directions:

Combine lemon juice, simple syrup, Jack Daniele's Tennessee rye into a shaker with ice and shake it.

Strain into a glass over fresh ice

Make the wine float on top

Take the orange together with the cherry and use it to garnish

Serve while chilled

Apple Cider Punch

Preparation time: 10 minutes

Servings: 5

Ingredients:

4 to 6 cups apple cider

1 cup applejack or Calvados

Pinch of ground cloves

1 cup Irish whiskey

Garnish: 1 red Delicious apple, halved and sliced thin, and 1 lime, sliced

1/4 cup fresh lime juice, strained

Directions:

Mix apple cider, lime juice, whiskey, and applejack in a punch bowl. Add in cloves and stir. Refrigerate for 1 hour. Fill in ice cubes or a block of ice. Use lime slices and apples to decorate the punch.

Cameron's Kick

Preparation time: 10 minutes

Servings: 1

Ingredients:

3/4 oz. Scotch whiskey

3/4 oz. Irish whiskey

1/2 tbsp. lemon juice

1/2 tbsp. orgeat syrup (or 2 dashes of orange bitters)

3 or 4 ice cubes

Directions:

In a cocktail shaker, mix all ingredients and shake forcefully. Transfer into a cocktail glass through a strainer.

Dirty Irishman

Preparation time: 4 minutes

Servings: 2

Ingredients:

1 (1.5 fluid oz.) jigger Irish cream liqueur

1 (1.5 fluid oz.) jigger Irish whiskey

Directions:

Fill ice into a short glass then add in Irish whiskey and Irish cream liqueur. Stir and serve.

Espresso old fashioned

Preparation time: 10 minutes

Servings: 2

Ingredients:

60ml redemption rye whiskey

Lemon twist

60ml espresso or cold-brew coffee

7.5ml simple syrup

1 dash Peychaud's bitters

1 dash Absinthe

Directions:

Place a dash of absinthe in a glass

Pour rye whiskey, espresso, simple syrup into a glass and mix with ice

Prepare a glass with an ice cube and strain over it.

Squeeze oil from a lemon twist and prepare it as garnish.

Serve

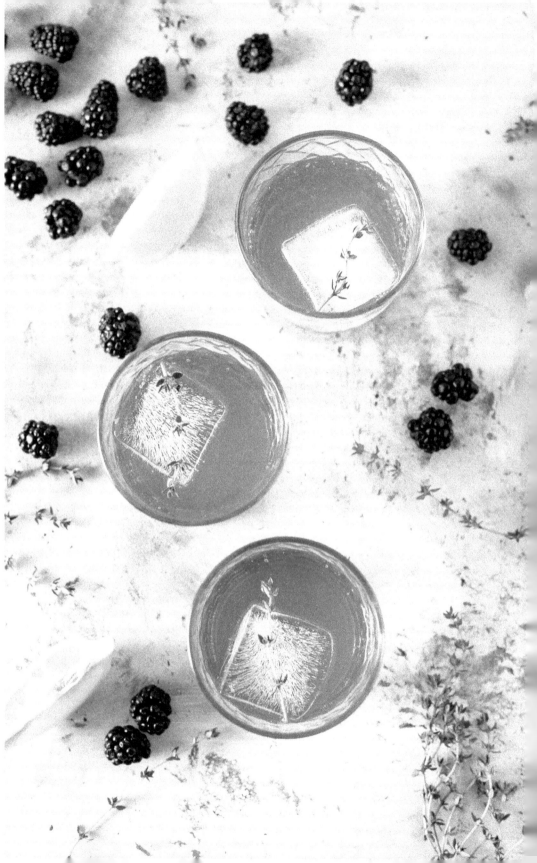

Tequila Cocktails

Galentine Cocktail

Preparation time: 5 minutes

Servings: 3

Ingredients:

1 cup pink lemonade

¼ cup lemon-lime soda

¼ cup fresh lemon juice

½ cup triple sec

1 cup tequila

Lemon slices, garnish

Ice

Directions:

Stir together pink lemonade, lemon-lime soda, lemon juice, triple sec, and tequila in a large pitcher with ice.

Pour into glasses and garnish with lemon slices.

Tequila Cup

Preparation time: 10 minutes

Servings: 2

Ingredients:

½ ounce orange curaçao

1 strawberry, hulled

1½ ounces 1800 Silver tequila

3 cucumber half-wheels

3 mint leaves

3 ounces Fresh Sour

7-Up, as required

Optional fruit: peach, apple, pear, tangerine, berries, etc.

Directions:

Mix all of the ingredients in a cocktail shaker with ice.

Shake casually and pour contents into a big glass.

Top with a splash of 7-Up.

Serve with a straw.

Agave Punch

Preparation time: 10 minutes

Servings: 2

Ingredients:

1 cup water

1 ounce triple sec

2 ounces pure agave reposado tequila

6 ounces frozen limeade concentrate

Lime half-wheels, for decoration (not necessary)

Directions:

Mix all of the ingredients apart from the lime half-wheel in a blender with four to 5 ice cubes.

Blend until the desired smoothness is achieved.

The mixture should not be too thick.

Pour into little cups and decorate each with a lime half-wheel.

Red Pepper Sangrita

Preparation time: 10 minutes

Servings: 1

Ingredients:

1½ ounces pure agave silver tequila

2½ ounces Pepper Mix (see below)

Whole red chili pepper, for decoration

Directions:

Mix the Pepper Mix and tequila in a cocktail shaker with ice.

Stir thoroughly (about ten seconds), strain into a chilled martini glass, and decorate with the red chili pepper.

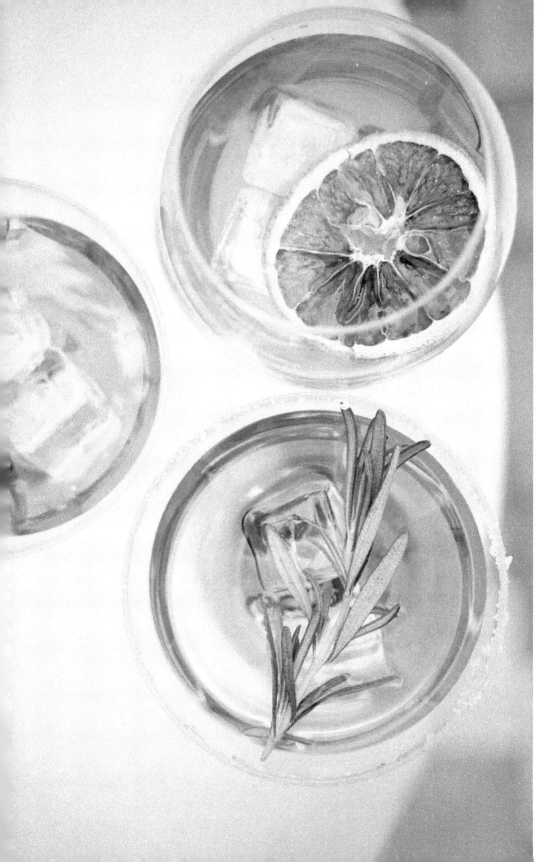

Rum Keto Cocktails

Blueberry Mojito

Preparation time: 10 minutes

Servings: 2

Ingredients:

3 lemons, chopped

350 ml (11.8 oz.) white rum

100 g (3.4 oz.) blueberries

600 ml (20.2 oz.) sparkling water

2 bruised mint sprigs, with leaves

2 tbsp granulated sugar

Directions:

In a jar, muddle the lemons, blueberries, and sugar together to get a syrup-like mixture.

Add the mint leaves and some ice cubes to the jar.

Pour the water and the rum, and stir everything together.

Strawberry Mojito

Preparation time: 10 minutes

Servings: 2

Ingredients:

350 ml (11.8oz.) white rum

2 limes, chopped

600 ml (20.3 oz.) sparkling water

Black pepper

2 tbsp granulated sugar

Ice cubes

2 mint sprigs, with leaves

10 strawberries

Directions:

In a jug, mix the strawberries, sugar, and limes until you get a creamy texture.

Bruise some mint leaves and add to the strawberry mixture, along with some black pepper.

Stir in the sparkling water and the rum.

Serve with ice cubes.

Sangrum

Preparation time: 10 minutes

Servings: 2

Ingredients:

½ cup chopped pineapple

½ cup light rum

1 apple, cored and cut

1 bottle of red wine

1 lemon, cut into wheels

1 liter 7-Up

1 pint strawberries, hulled and cut

12 whole cloves

2 limes, cut into wheels

2 oranges, cut into wedges

Directions:

Stick the cloves in the orange wedges or apple slices.

Mix the orange wedges and apple slices with all of the rest of the ingredients except the 7-Up in a big ceramic or glass container and stir thoroughly.

Cover and place in your fridge for a minimum of 4 hours (preferably overnight).

Just before you serve, put in the 7-Up.

Serve over ice.

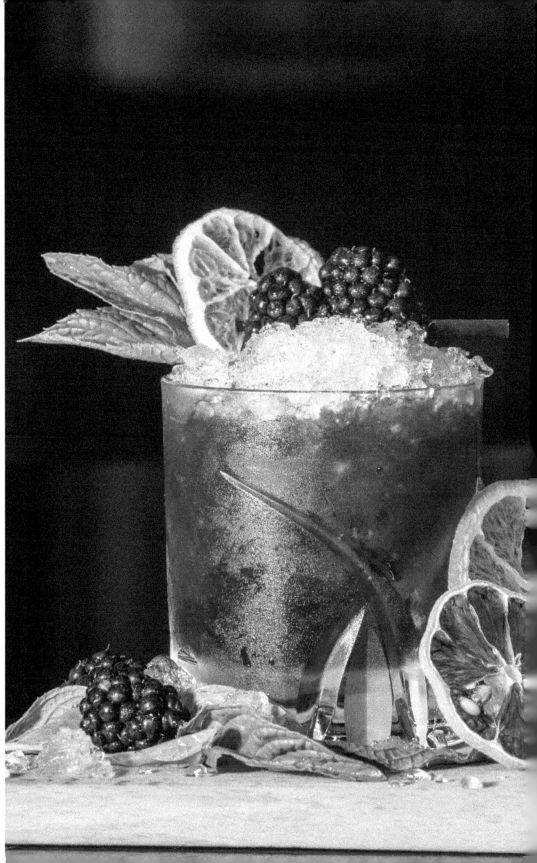

Vodka Keto Cocktails

Woo Woo

Preparation time: 10 minutes

Servings: 2

Ingredients:

100 ml (3.4 oz.) cranberry juice

50 ml (1.7 oz.) vodka

The juice of ½ lemon

24 ml (0.8 oz.) peach schnapps

Ice cubes

Lime wedges

Directions:

Put all the liquid ingredients, the lime juice, and some ice into your cocktail shaker, and shake well.

Strain the cocktail into a tumbler, and add additional ice.

Garnish with lime wedges before serving.

Sex on The Beach

Preparation time: 10 minutes

Servings: 2

Ingredients:

50 ml (1.7 oz.) vodka

50 ml (1.7 oz.) cranberry juice

25 ml (0.85 oz.) peach schnapps

The juice of 2 oranges

Glacé cherries to garnish

Ice cubes

Orange slices, to garnish

Directions:

Fill the glasses with ice cubes.

Pour the fruit juices, vodka, and peach schnapps into a large jug. Stir everything together.

Pour the mixture into the two glasses and stir once again.

Garnish with the cherries and additional orange slices before serving.

Bloody Mary

Preparation time: 10 minutes

Servings: 2

Ingredients:

200 ml (6.7 oz.) tomato juice

1 tsp sherry vinegar

50 ml (1.7 oz.) vodka

Ice cubes

2 tbsp amontillado sherry

A pinch of salt

Tabasco, to taste

Worcestershire sauce, to taste

Lemon juice

Celery sticks, to garnish

Lemon wedges, to garnish

Pepper, to serve (optional)

Directions:

Pour the vodka, tomato juice, sherry vinegar, and amontillado into a tall glass along with some ice cubes.

Season with Tabasco, celery salt, and Worcestershire sauce. Add lemon juice to taste.

Serve with lemon wedges, celery sticks, and freshly ground black (optional).

Long Island Iced Tea

Preparation time: 10 minutes

Servings: 2

Ingredients:

50 ml (1.7 oz.) London dry gin

50 ml (1.7 oz.) vanilla vodka

50 ml (1.7 oz.) tequila

50 ml (1.7 oz.) triple sec

50 ml (1.7 oz.) rum

50 ml (1.7 oz.) fresh lime juice

500 ml (17 oz.) cola

2 limes, cut into wedges

Ice cubes

Directions:

Pour all the spirits and liqueur into a large jug. Add lime juice.

Fill ½ of the jug with ice cubes and stir well.

Fill the jug with cola and stir once again.

Add the lime wedges and serve the cocktail into 4 tall glasses with additional ice cubes.

Espresso Martini

Preparation time: 10 minutes

Servings: 2

Ingredients:

100 ml (3.4 oz.) vodka

100 g (3.4 oz.) golden caster syrup

50 ml (1.7 oz.) coffee liqueur

50 ml (1.7 oz.) freshly brewed espresso

A few coffee beans, to garnish

Directions:

Bring the caster sugar to boil in 50 ml (1.7 oz.) of water. Allow the mixture to cool, stirring frequently until you obtain the right consistency for your sugar syrup.

Pour 1 tbsp of this sugar into a cocktail shaker with all the other ingredients.

Shake well and serve into 2 refrigerated martini glasses.

Garnish with additional coffee beans.

Caipiroska

Preparation time: 5 minutes

Servings: 2

Ingredients:

2 oz. vodka

¾ oz. sugar syrup

Ice

Lime

Directions:

Place 2 lime wedges into a rocks glass and muddle

Fill a rocks glass to the top with ice

Pour in ¾ oz. of sugar syrup and 2 oz. of vodka

Stir gently

Top up with crushed ice

Garnish with lemon slices

Cape Codder

Preparation time: 5 minutes

Servings: 5

Ingredients:

2 oz. vodka

5 oz. cranberry juice

Ice

Cranberry, for garnish

Lime wedge or mint, for garnish

Directions:

Fill a highball glass to the top with ice

Pour in 2 oz. of vodka

Garnish with cranberries and lime or mint

Cosmopolitan

Preparation time: 10 minutes

Servings: 2

Ingredients:

1½ oz. vodka

¾ oz. triple sec liqueur

2 oz. cranberry juice

¼ oz. lime juice

Orange zest, for garnish

Lime slice, for garnish

Ice

Directions:

Pour 1½ oz. of vodka into a shaker, ¾ oz. of triple sec liqueur, ¼ oz. of lime juice, and 2 oz. of cranberry juice

Fill the shaker with ice cubes and shake

Use a culinary torch to flambee the oils from the orange zest over the cocktail after straining in a chilled glass

Rim the sides of the glass with flamed orange zest, put it in the glass, and garnish with a slice of lime

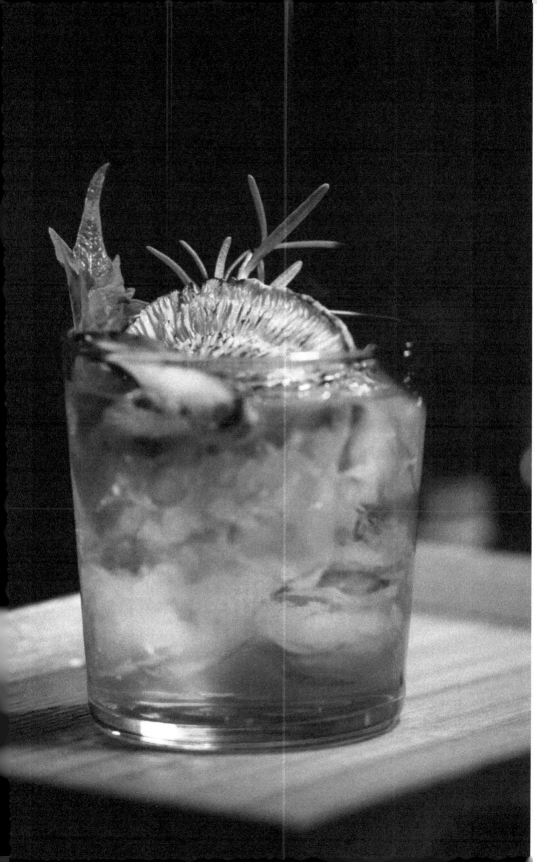

Keto Liqueurs

Coffee liqueur

Preparation time: 60 minutes

Servings: 3

Ingredients:

15.8oz. of mocha coffee or espresso

15.8oz. of sugar

Alcohol

Directions:

To prepare the Coffee Liqueur, start by preparing the coffee with the mocha (or if you prefer with the coffee machine,) which you will pour into a pan with high edges. Add the sugar and light the very low heat to melt it.

To facilitate the operation, you can mix with a spatula or with a wooden spoon. When the sugar is completely dissolved, pour the mixture into a small bowl to cool.

When it is well cooled, add the alcohol and mix it carefully with the other ingredients.

Finally, distribute Coffee Liqueur in new or well-washed glass bottles, perfectly clean and dried (once washed, it is advisable to dry them upside down on a clean towel). Screw the cap on and close the bottles tightly so that no air enters. Let Coffee

Liqueur rest in the bottles for at least 2 weeks before consuming it.

Cherry liqueur

Preparation time: 2 days

Servings: 3

Ingredients:

14.1oz. of pitted cherries

14.1oz. of pure alcohol (~95°)

18.3oz. of water

3.3oz. of sugar

Directions:

To prepare Cherry Liqueur, first, wash and dry the cherries. Add the cherries to a glass jar, add the alcohol, close with the lid and leave to macerate at room temperature for a week.

After the maceration time, take the jar again, filter the mixture through a strainer and collect the infusion in a container. Pour sugar into a saucepan.

Add the water and heat the syrup over medium heat for 15 minutes. Let the syrup cool slightly, then add it to the infusion.

Mix in the Liqueur obtained, pour it into a jar with an airtight seal, and let it rest for 3 weeks at room temperature. After this time, your Cherry Liqueur will be ready: pour it in a bottle and keep it at room temperature, if it is not too hot, or place it in the refrigerator.

Tips:

Cherry Liqueur can be kept for 90 days in the refrigerator or at room temperature if it is not too hot. Once opened, it is preferable to keep it in the refrigerator.

If you like an extra aromatic touch, add vanilla seeds, cinnamon sticks, or orange zest to your liqueur.

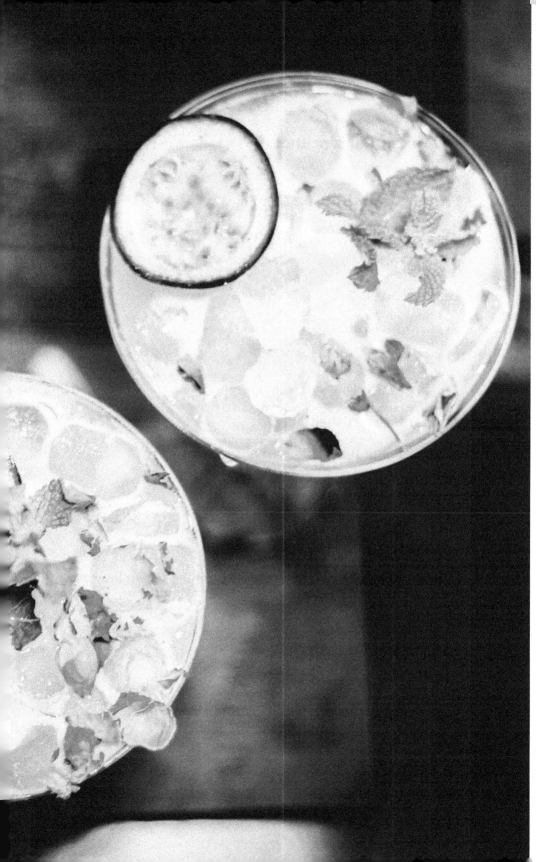

Keto Mocktails

Mint Julep Mocktail

Preparation time: 60 minutes

Servings: 3

Ingredients:

¼ cup water (filtered)

¼ cup of sugar, white

1 tbsp. of mint leaves (fresh, chopped)

2 cups of ice (crushed)

½ cup of lemonade (ready-made)

For Garnishing:

Fresh sprigs of mint

Directions:

Combine filtered water, white sugar, and 1 tbsp. chopped mint leaves. Stir, bring to boil.

Cook mixture until sugar is dissolved. Remove from heat. Set aside for cooling.

After an hour or so, strain the mint leaves out.

Fill two cups with crushed ice. Add half lemonade in each cup. Top with a splash of sugar syrup.

Garnish cups with straw and sprig of mint. Serve.

Arnold Palmer

Preparation time: 5 minutes

Servings: 3

Ingredients:

2 parts of iced tea for each

1 part of lemonade for each

For garnishing:

slices of lemon

Directions:

Pour iced tea and lemonade into two ice-filled tall glasses.

Stir thoroughly.

Garnish with lemon slices. Serve.

Raspberry-Cranberry Twist

Preparation time: 10 minutes

Servings: 3

Ingredients:

1 x 12 fluid oz. bottle or can of carbonated beverage (lemon-lime flavor)

12 fluid oz. of cranberry-raspberry juice

Directions:

Mix the lemon-lime soda with cranberry-raspberry juice. Pour it over ice. Serve.

Sweet Virgin Sunrise

Preparation time: 5 minutes

Servings: 3

Ingredients:

4 fluid oz. of orange juice (fresh-squeezed if possible)

Ice

½ fluid oz. of grenadine

Orange slice for garnishing

Directions:

Pour ice into a highball glass and add the orange juice.

Pour grenadine slowly over juice.

Use an orange slice to garnish and serve.

Chicha Morada

Preparation time: 5hour

Servings: 3

Ingredients:

1 (3½ pound) fresh pineapple

2 Granny Smith apples (cored)

1 (16 ounce) bag dried purple corn

2 (2") sticks of cinnamon

½ tsp whole cloves

¾ cup packed light brown sugar

7 pints water

½ cup + 2 tbsp freshly squeezed lemon juice

½ cup + 2 tbsp freshly squeezed lime juice

1 tsp kosher salt

Wheels of fresh lime (to garnish)

Ice (to serve)

Directions:

Trim, peel, and core the pineapple. Set the peel and core to one side.

Dice ¼ of the diced pineapple (approximately 1 cup) and set the remaining aside for alternative use.

Cut one of the cored apples into quarters.

In a large size pan, combine the pineapple peel, pineapple core, and apple with the corn, cinnamon stick, cloves, brown sugar, and 7 pints of water).

Cover the pan with a lid and over moderate-high heat, bring to boil.

Remove the lid, and turn the heat down to moderate. Simmer the corn until it softens and the liquid slightly reduces, for approximately 60 minutes.

With a slotted spoon, remove any solids and discard them.

Pour the liquid through a strainer into a large size heat-safe bowl and allow it to stand for 45 minutes, or until it no longer steams.

Whisk in the fresh lemon juice followed by the lime juice and salt, and transfer to the fridge for 2 hours, until cold.

Peel the remaining apple and dice.

Add the diced apple and diced pineapple to a punch bowl or large pitcher.

Pour the Chicha Morada over the fruit, garnish with wheels of fresh lime, and serve with ice.

Mint watermelon

Preparation time: 10 minutes

Servings: 4

Ingredients:

1/2 cup cold-pressed watermelon juice

1 tablespoon. freshly squeezed lime

2 mint leaves

fresh mint for garnish

lime zest for garnish

Directions:

Pour all the ingredients into a shaker with a handful of ice. Shake for 30 seconds to 1 minute.

Garnish with fresh mint and lime zest.

Serve on ice.

Peach and rosemary iced tea

Preparation time: 10 minutes

Servings: 4

Ingredients:

1 dl of water

75 g of sugar

200 g of diced peaches

For the mocktail:

¾ of a liter of water

1 Earl Gray Everton teabag

3 sprigs of rosemary

½ lemon

½ peach in wedges

Directions:

Boil the water with the sugar in a saucepan. Add the peaches and cook for about 10 minutes. Now, remove from the heat and let the syrup flavor for about an hour.

Meanwhile, boil the tea water and let our Earl Gray with rosemary infuse for about 15 minutes. Remove the sachets and the rosemary and add the peach syrup and the juice of ½ lemon. Let it cool and put everything in the refrigerator for about 1 hour. Serve it to your guests with peach wedges, rosemary, and ice cubes.

Raspberry Splash

Preparation time: 10 minutes

Servings: 4

Ingredients:

4 dl of water

2 Earl Gray Everton teabags

½ file

3 dl of ginger ale

8 sprigs of mint

80 g of raspberries

to taste ice cubes

Directions:

Bring the water to a boil and add the Earl Gray sachets, leaving to infuse for about 5 minutes. Squeeze the lime and mix the juice with the cooled black tea and ginger ale.

Spread the mint, raspberries, and ice cubes in 4 glasses. Pour in the tea and voila… your mocktail is ready to serve.

Not a Hot Toddy

Preparation time: 10 minutes

Servings: 1

Ingredients:

1 tablespoon organic honey

1 teaspoon fresh orange juice

½ teaspoon ground nutmeg

½ teaspoon cloves

½ teaspoon grated cinnamon

7 ounces hot tea

Orange wedge for garnish

Directions:

Add honey, orange juice, and spices to the warmed mug.

Top with the fresh-brewed, hot tea. Stir well to combine.

Use an orange wedge to garnish and serve.

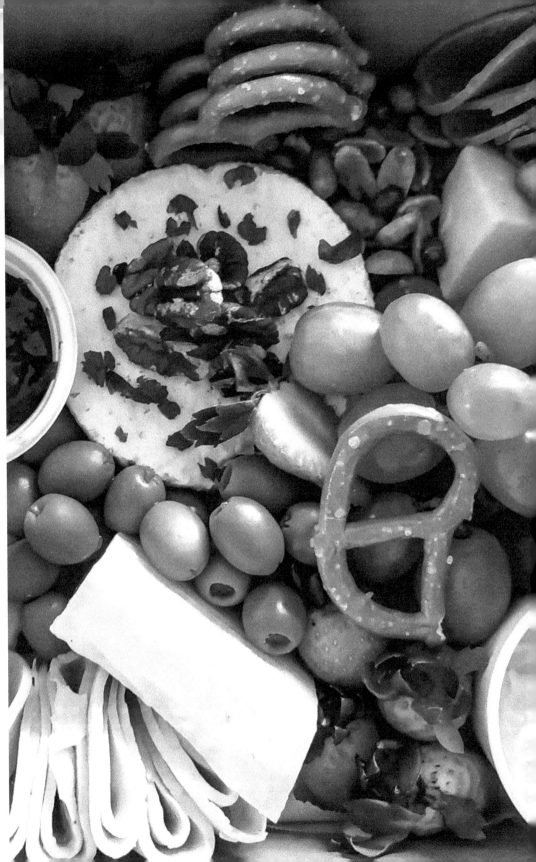

Mushroom and Asparagus Frittata

Preparation time: 10 minutes

Cooking Time: 45 minutes

Servings: 8

Ingredients:

8 large eggs

1/2 cup of ricotta cheese

2 tbsps. of lemon juice

1/2 tsp. of salt

1/4 tsp. of pepper

1 tbsp. of olive oil

8 ounces of asparagus spears

1 onion (sliced)

1/3 cup of sweet green pepper

3/4 cup of Portobello mushrooms (sliced)

Directions:

Preheat your oven at one hundred and fifty degrees Celsius. Combine ricotta cheese, eggs, pepper, lemon juice, and salt in a bowl. Heat oil in an iron skillet. Add onion, asparagus, mushrooms, and red pepper. Cook for eight minutes. Remove the asparagus from the skillet.

Cut the spears of asparagus into pieces of two-inch. Return the spears to the skillet. Add the mixture of eggs. Bake in the oven for twenty minutes. Let the frittata sit for five minutes.

Cut the frittata into wedges. Serve warm.

Nutrition: calories 200, fat 8, fiber 4, carbs 8, protein 3

Sausage Balls

Preparation time: 10 minutes

Cooking Time: 45 minutes

Servings: 6

Ingredients:

1 pound of spicy pork sausage (ground)

8 ounces of cream cheese

1/2 cup of cheddar cheese (shredded)

1/3 cup of parmesan cheese (shredded)

1 tbsp. of Dijon mustard

1/2 tsp. of garlic powder

1/4 tsp. of salt

Directions:

Preheat your oven at one hundred and seventy degrees Celsius. Use parchment paper for lining a baking sheet.

Combine cream cheese, sausage, parmesan cheese, cheddar cheese, garlic powder, mustard, and salt in a mixing bowl. Mix well.

Take one tbsp. of the mixture. Roll it into a ball. Repeat for the remaining mixture. Arrange the prepared balls on the lined baking tray. Bake for thirty minutes.

Serve hot.

Nutrition: calories 110, fat 10, fiber 1, carbs 3, protein 6

Ranch Cauliflower Crackers

Preparation time: 10 minutes

Cooking Time: 30 minutes

Servings: 6

Ingredients:

12 ounces of cauliflower rice

Cheesecloth

1 large egg

1 tbsp. of ranch salad dressing mix (dry)

1/8 tsp. of cayenne pepper

1 cup of parmesan cheese (shredded)

Directions:

Add the cauliflower rice to a large bowl. Microwave for four minutes covered. Transfer the cauliflower rice to a strainer lined with cheesecloth. Squeeze out excess moisture. Preheat the oven to two hundred degrees Celsius. Use parchment paper for lining a baking tray.

Combine egg, cauliflower rice, ranch mix, and pepper in a bowl. Add the cheese. Mix well. Take two tbsps. Of the mixture and add them to the baking tray. Flatten with your hands. The thinner you can make the mixture; the crispier will be the crackers.

Bake for ten minutes. Flip the crackers. Bake for ten minutes. Serve warm.

Nutrition: calories 110, fat 10, fiber 1, carbs 3, protein 6

Pork Belly Cracklings

Preparation time: 10 minutes

Cooking Time: 80 minutes

Servings: 6

Ingredients:

3 pounds of pork belly (with skin)

2 cups of water

4 tbsps. of Cajun seasoning

Directions:

Keep the pork belly in the refrigerator for forty minutes. Cut the pork into cubes of a three-fourth inch. Fill a cast-iron pot with one-fourth portion of water. Add one tsp. of Cajun seasoning. Boil the water.

Add the cubes of pork belly. Cook for twenty minutes. Cover the pot once fat begins to pop and sizzle. Cook for fifteen minutes. Drain the pork cracklings.

Sprinkle remaining seasoning from the top. Serve immediately.

Nutrition: calories 383, fat 14, fiber 4, carbs 3, protein 8

Keto Berry Mousse

Preparation time: 5 minutes

Cooking Time: 0 minutes

Servings: 2

Ingredients:

2 cups heavy whipping cream

3 oz. fresh raspberries

2 oz. chopped pecans

½ lemon, zested

¼ tsp vanilla extract

Directions:

Beat cream in a bowl using a hand mixer until it forms peaks.

Stir in vanilla and lemon zest and mix well until incorporated.

Fold in nuts and berries and mix well.

Cover the mixture with plastic wrap and refrigerate for 3 hours.

Serve fresh.

Nutrition: Calories: 254 Fat: 9 g Cholesterol: 13 mg Sodium: 179 mg Protein 7.5 g

Peanut Butter Mousse

Preparation time: 5 minutes

Cooking Time: 0 minutes

Servings: 4

Ingredients:

½ cup heavy whipping cream

4 oz. cream cheese, softened

¼ cup natural peanut butter

¼ cup powdered Swerve sweetener

½ tsp vanilla extract

Directions:

Beat ½ cup cream in a medium bowl with a hand mixer until it forms peaks.

Beat cream cheese with peanut butter in another bowl until creamy.

Stir in vanilla, a pinch of salt, and sweetener to the peanut butter mix and combine until smooth.

Fold in the prepared whipped cream and mix well until fully incorporated.

Divide the mousse into 4 serving glasses.

Garnish as desired.

Nutrition: Calories: 290 Fat: 21.5 Cholesterol: 12 Sodium: 9
Protein: 6

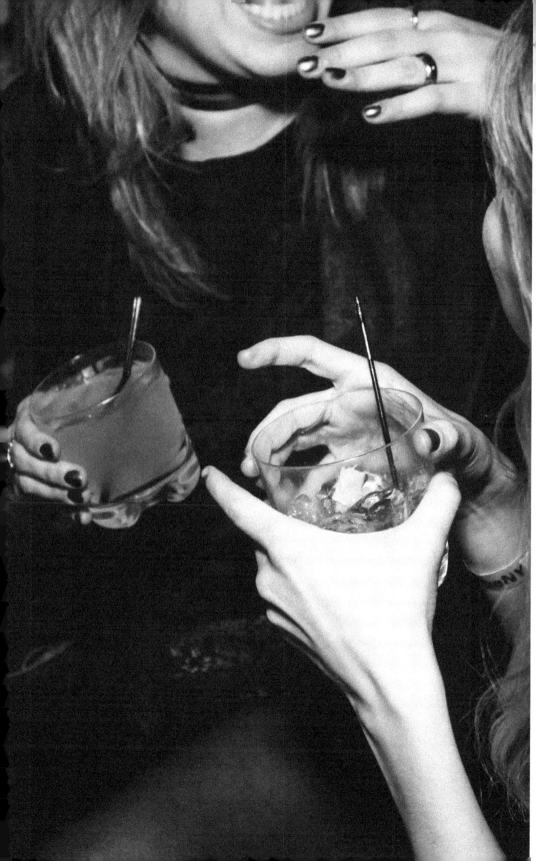

Conclusion

This book will help you kickstart your fitness journey and ultimately support you in reaching your ideal body weight. Start by understanding how Keto Cocktail works and choose a cocktail that suits your needs. Find out which drinks you can drink and which ones you should avoid, calculate your macros, plan your meals and make a list of food items you need to buy. To increase results, incorporate some form of exercise every day. It could be a 30 minute walk or a high intensity training session. Whatever you do never give up live your keto life!

Keto Alcohol Drinks

Easy Keto Cocktails Recipes for Beginners you Can Enjoy at Home with Your Friends to Lose Weight and Burn Fat

Jenny Kern

Introduction

Thank you for purchasing this book. So, you've had a long, tiring day at the office and are mentally and physically drained. The only thing on your mind right now is to crawl into your favorite bar, say hello to your usual bartender, and order a nice and tasty cocktail to help you kick back and unwind. For years, cocktails, those delicious alcoholic blends, have been helping tense and stressed people relax and unwind. However, how many of these drinkers know how to make them themselves? In this book we will follow you step by step to create your favorite cocktails. I hope you like them.

Enjoy.

Wine and Champagne Keto Cocktails

Lava Champagne with Gelatin

Preparation time: 10 minutes

Servings: 6

Ingredients:

1 750-ml. bottle champagne

1 c. vodka

1 c. boiling water

1 3-oz. package blue or red instant Jell-O mix

Directions:

Mix the boiling water and gelatin mix in a bowl for around two minutes or until the mixture completely dissolves.

Pour in the vodka. Pour this liquid mixture into individual portions or small paper cups. Chill in the fridge for approximately two hours or until set.

Once the gelatin mixture is set, pour the champagne into cocktail glasses. Use a fork to break up the gelatin.

Add the mixture to a glass of champagne. Stir it gradually to produce some lava action. Serve and enjoy.

Raspberry cocktail

Preparation time: 10 minutes

Servings: 4

Ingredients:

2 bottles of cold sparkling wine of excellent quality, if you like you can choose it more or less sweet

4 spoons of sugar

4 little boxes of fresh raspberries, or an equivalent quantity of frozen raspberries

Directions:

Pour the wine, which, as mentioned, must be very cold, into a decorative container, for example, a crystal or silver bowl. Pour in the sugar, and give it a stir. Add the raspberries.

Serve as an aperitif, using a silver ladle to pour in cups or flutes.

Bishop Cocktail

Preparation time: 10 minutes

Servings: 3

Ingredients:

30 milliliters orange juice

2 teaspoons runny honey

75 milliliters tawny port wine

90 milliliters boiling water

7 cloves

Directions:

Use preheated heat-proof glass. Muddle cloves in the base of the shaker. Put in boiling water and stir in honey and other ingredients. Strain into glass. Use grated nutmeg to garnish.

Orange punch

Preparation time: 30 minutes

Servings: 4

Ingredients:

4 cups of water

25oz. of sugar

3 cups of Aperol

3 untreated oranges

Directions:

To prepare the punch, wash and dry the oranges well, peel them with the help of a peeler, then keep the peel aside.

Cut fruit in half and squeeze them using a juicer, then strain the juice and put it in a large bowl.

Prepare the syrup now: in a saucepan, heat the sugar with the water, and cook everything over low heat until the sugar has completely dissolved. Meanwhile, add Aperol to the orange juice.

When ready, add the sugar syrup. Finally, add the orange peel (which you had previously kept aside) and leave to infuse for a few minutes. Serve the punch still hot.

Tips:

Store the punch in the refrigerator, closed in an airtight container, for a maximum of 3-4 days. When serving, heat it in a saucepan.

Frozen peach champagne cocktail

Preparation time: 10 minutes

Servings: 4

Ingredients:

4ml of Alize peach

1 cup ice

12ml chilled champagne

3 tablespoons powdered sugar

2 cups frozen peach slices

2 tablespoons grenadine

Directions:

Mix frozen peaches, powdered sugar, Alize peach, and ice in a blender. Blend the mixture and add champagne until it smoothens

Pour in the remaining champagne and stir it thoroughly

Place in each glass ¼ of the mixture then take a tablespoon of grenadine and add to each of the glasses. On top add the remaining peach mixture

Garnish then serve.

Basil and Pomegranate Champagne Cocktail

Preparation time: 10 minutes

Servings: 4

Ingredients:

2 fresh basil leaves

4-fl. oz. champagne

1 tbsp. pomegranate juice

Directions:

Put the basil leaves in the bottom of the champagne flute. Add the pomegranate juice.

Muddle the leaves lightly to release their flavor. Top the mixture with champagne. Serve.

Peach Blossom Champagne

Preparation time: 10 minutes

Servings: 8

Ingredients:

2/3 c. peach schnapps

5 c. orange juice

2 c. ice cubes

1 tbsp. grenadine syrup

1 ½ c. champagne, chilled

Optional ingredient: 6 peach slices

Directions:

Mix peach schnapps and orange juice in a pitcher. Place in your fridge for around thirty minutes or until chilled.

Pour a half-cup of the mixture into 6 glasses. Add around two to three ice cubes into each glass.

Add three to four tablespoons of champagne per glass. Drizzle a half teaspoon of the grenadine syrup into each glass. Do not stir. If you are using peach slices, garnish each drink with one slice. Serve.

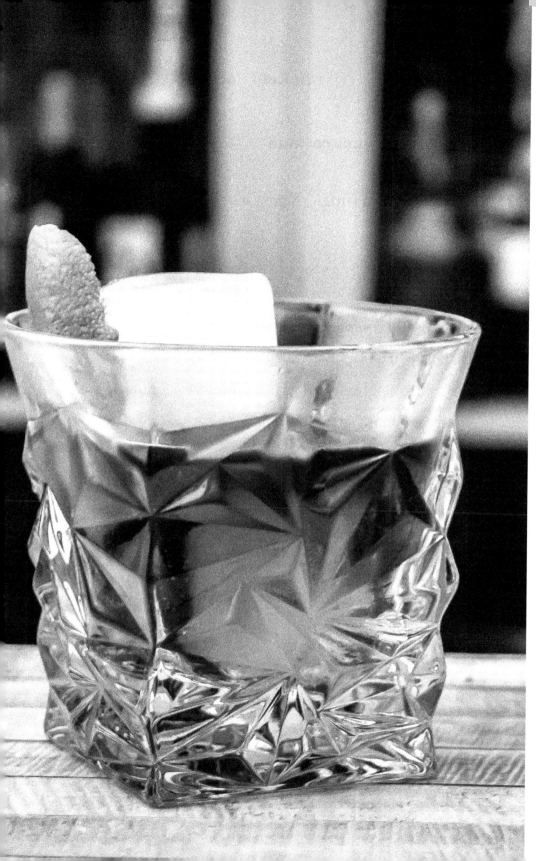

Gin Keto Cocktails

Orange juice cocktail

Preparation time: 10 minutes

Servings: 6

Ingredients:

4 cups of Prosecco or Spumante Brut

1/2 cup of gin

1/2 cup of natural orange juice from fresh oranges

2 teaspoons of sugar (optional)

Directions:

Squeeze the oranges.

Divide the juice into cold cocktail glasses (preferably flute or hurricane), passing it directly through a colander.

Then add the Spumante Brut or Prosecco.

Also, add the gin in the 6 glasses, if you want - add the sugar, mix, and serve.

Tips:

You can decorate the glass with orange slices and dip a cherry in alcohol.

Champagne pink cocktail

Preparation time: 15 minutes

Servings: 2

Calories: 109 Kcal

Ingredients:

2 pieces of candied ginger

0.5oz. of sugar

2 tablespoons of fruit and ginger syrup

1 cup of very cold rosé champagne

6oz. of mixed candied fruit

2 cups of water

5 tablespoons of orange vodka

ice cubes to taste

Directions:

Prepare the fruit and ginger syrup in advance.

Bring the water to a boil, then throw in the candied fruit, ginger, and sugar.

Simmer gently for 5 minutes, then let cool.

Blend everything with a powerful mixer until a homogeneous mixture is obtained.

Pass through a sieve and refrigerate in an air-tight container until ready to use.

To prepare the cocktail, pour the vodka, the mixture obtained, and two tablespoons of syrup into a shaker filled with ice. Shake with energy.

Fill two flutes with champagne and then complete them with the contents of the shaker passed through the strainer. Serve immediately.

Devil Twister

Preparation time: 10 minutes

Servings: 2

Ingredients:

8 milliliters Fernet Branca

8 milliliters triple sec

15 milliliters cold water

15 milliliters Dubonnet Red

60 milliliters London dry gin

Directions:

Shake ingredients with ice and strain into chilled glass. Garnish using lemon zest twist.

Destiny

Preparation time: 10 minutes

Servings: 2

Ingredients:

8 milliliters lemon juice

8 milliliters sugar syrup

15 milliliters crème de cassis

15 milliliters vanilla liqueur

30 milliliters London dry gin

90 milliliters cranberry juice

6 fresh blackberries

Directions:

Muddle blackberries in the base of the shaker. Put in other ingredients, shake with ice, and strain into a glass filled with crushed ice. Garnish using mint.

Crash Impact

Preparation time: 10 minutes

Servings: 2

Ingredients:

8 milliliters triple sec

15 milliliters dry vermouth

15 milliliters sweet vermouth8 milliliters lemon juice

2 dashes bitters

60 milliliters London dry gin

Directions:

Shake ingredients with ice and strain into chilled glass. Garnish using maraschino cherry.

Country Breeze

Preparation time: 10 minutes

Servings: 2

Ingredients:

15 milliliters crème de cassis

60 milliliters London dry gin

105 milliliters apple juice

Directions:

Shake ingredients with ice and strain into ice-filled glass. Garnish using strawberries and blueberries.

Alexander Cocktail

Preparation time: 10 minutes

Servings: 2

Ingredients:

15 milliliters whipping cream

30 milliliters white crème de cacao liqueur

60 milliliters London dry gin

Directions:

Shake ingredients with ice and strain into chilled glass. Garnish using grated nutmeg.

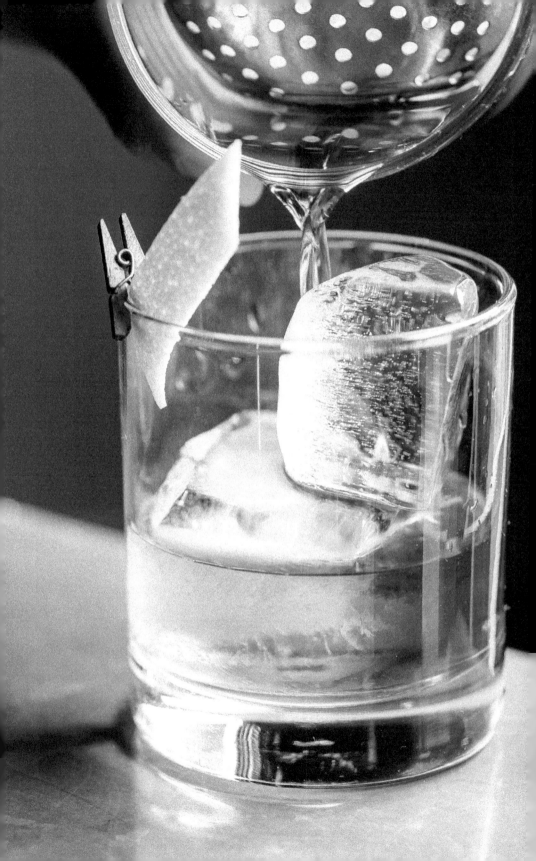

Whiskey Keto Cocktails

Original Irish Cream

Preparation time: 15 minutes

Servings: 12

Ingredients:

1 cup heavy cream

1 (14 oz.) can sweetened condensed milk

1 2/3 cups Irish whiskey

1 tsp. instant coffee granules

2 tbsps. chocolate syrup

1 tsp. vanilla extract

1 tsp. almond extract

Directions:

Mix almond extract, vanilla extract, chocolate syrup, instant coffee, Irish whiskey, sweetened condensed milk, and heavy cream in a blender.

Blend for 20-30 seconds on the high setting.

Keep in a tightly sealed container in the fridge. Shake thoroughly before serving.

St. Michael's Irish Americano

Preparation time: 10 minutes

Servings: 2

Ingredients:

2 (1.5 fluid oz.) jiggers espresso coffee

2 (1.5 fluid oz.) jiggers Irish whiskey

1 tbsp. white sugar

1 tbsp. heavy cream

6 fluid oz. hot water

2 tbsps. whipped cream, garnish

Directions:

In your favorite mug, pour the espresso in then put in hot water, tbsp. cream, sugar, and Irish whiskey.

Use a dollop of whipped cream to garnish.

Shamrock

Preparation time: 10 minutes

Servings: 2

Ingredients:

15 milliliters cold water

15 milliliters green Chartreuse

15 milliliters green crème de menthe

45 milliliters dry vermouth

45 milliliters Irish whiskey

Directions:

Shake ingredients with ice and strain into chilled glass. Garnish using mint.

Rat Pack Manhattan

Preparation time: 10 minutes

Servings: 2

Ingredients:

15 milliliters Grand Marnier

22 milliliters dry vermouth

22 milliliters sweet vermouth

45 milliliters bourbon whiskey

3 dashes bitters

Directions:

Chill glass, add Grand Marnier, swirl to coat and then discard. Stir other ingredients with ice and strain into liqueur-coated glass. Garnish using orange zest twist and maraschino cherry.

Quebec

Preparation time: 10 minutes

Servings: 2

Ingredients:

2 dashes of orange bitters

60 milliliters Canadian whiskey

60 milliliters Dubonnet Red

Directions:

Stir ingredients and strain into chilled glass. Garnish using orange zest twist.

Tequila Cocktails

Sangrita

Preparation time: 10 minutes

Servings: 5

Ingredients:

¼ cup fresh lime juice

1 cup orange juice

2 cups tomato juice

2 teaspoons chopped onion

2 teaspoons hot sauce

2 teaspoons Worcestershire sauce

lime wedges, for serving

salt and freshly ground black pepper to taste

shot of pure agave tequila (a silver tequila is preferable because its agave bite complements the spicy sangrita)

Directions:

Mix the lime juice, onion, hot sauce, Worcestershire, and salt and pepper in a blender.

Blend until the desired smoothness is achieved.

In a pitcher, mix the mixed mixture with the orange juice and tomato juice.

Chill.

Before you serve, stir thoroughly, pour into little glasses, and pour tequila into separate shot glasses.

Drink the tequila, suck on a lime wedge, and chase it with the sangrita.

Mango Sangrita

Preparation time: 10 minutes

Servings: 2

Ingredients:

1 ounce Fresh Sour

1 ounce mango puree

1 teaspoon Tabasco

1½ ounces silver tequila

2 ounces tomato juice

Directions:

Mix all of the ingredients in a cocktail shaker with ice and stir contents.

Strain into a shot glass or martini glass.

Reverse Wind

Preparation time: 10 minutes

Servings: 2

Ingredients:

½ fresh egg white

15 milliliters maple syrup

22 milliliters lemon juice

2 dashes bitters

60 milliliters tequila

Directions:

Shake ingredients with ice and strain into chilled glass. Garnish using lemon zest twist.

Requiem Daiquiri

Preparation time: 10 minutes

Servings: 2

Ingredients:

8 milliliters navy rum

8 milliliters sugar syrup

15 milliliters lime juice

30 milliliters tequila

Directions:

Shake ingredients with ice and strain into chilled glass. Garnish using a lime wedge.

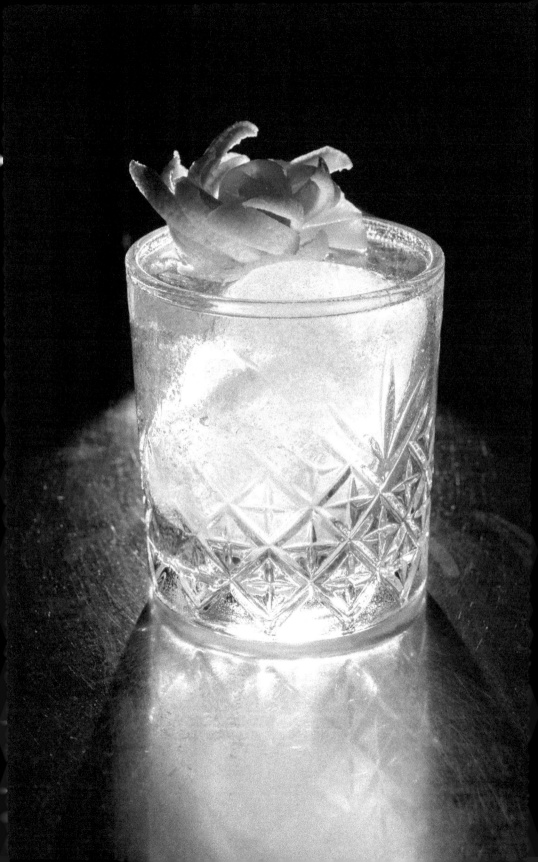

Rum Keto Cocktails

Piña colada

Preparation time: 10 minutes

Servings: 2

Ingredients:

60 ml (2 oz.) white rum

120 ml (4 oz.) pineapple juice

60 ml (2 oz.) coconut cream

Pineapple wedges, to garnish

Directions:

Process all the ingredients along with some ice in a blender, until you get a smooth texture.

Pour into a tall glass.

Garnish with some pineapple wedges.

Frozen Strawberry Daiquiri

Preparation time: 10 minutes

Servings: 6

Ingredients:

100 ml (3.4 oz.) rum

200 g (6.8 oz.) ice

500 g (17 oz.) strawberries

The juice of ½ lime

Lime slices, to garnish

1 strawberry, halved, to garnish

Directions:

Blend the strawberries until you get a creamy texture, and remove all seeds.

Put the puree into the blender with rum, lime juice, and ice.

Divide the blended mixture between 2 Martini glasses.

Garnish with lime slices and strawberry halves.

Apple Cooler

Preparation time: 5 minutes

Servings: 2

Ingredients:

2 oz. white rum

4 oz. apple juice

2 oz. Sprite

Ice

Apple, for garnish

Directions:

Fill a highball glass to the top with ice

Pour in 3 ½ oz. of apple juice and 1 ½ oz. of white rum

Top up with Sprite and stir gently

Garnish with 3 apple wedges

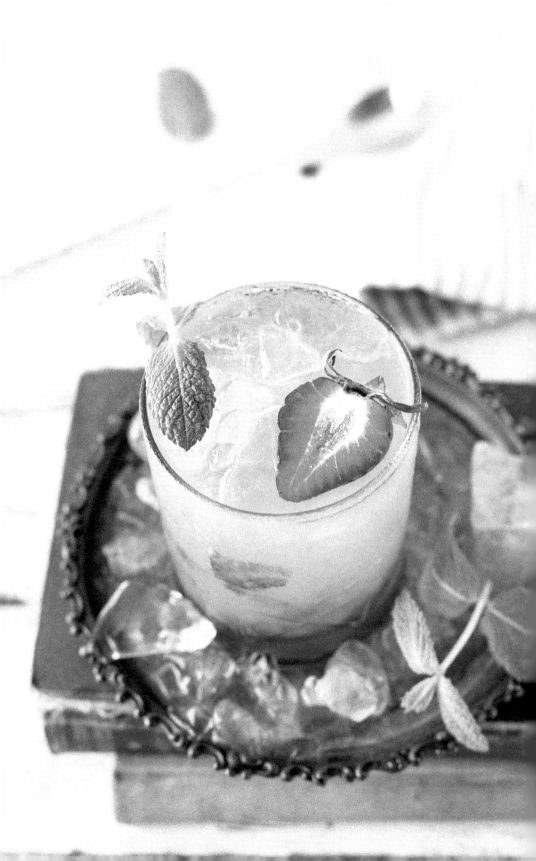

Vodka Keto Cocktails

Frozen special Martini

Preparation time: 10 minutes

Servings: 2

Ingredients:

1 oz. vodka

1 oz. coffee liqueur

1½ oz. espresso coffee

¼ oz. vanilla syrup

Ice

Coffee beans, for garnish

Directions:

Pour 1½ oz. of chilled espresso, ¼ oz. of vanilla syrup, 1 oz. of coffee liqueur, and 1 oz. of vodka into a shaker

Fill the shaker with ice cubes and shake

Garnish with coffee beans after straining in a chilled glass

Moscow Mule

Preparation time: 5 minutes

Servings: 2

Ingredients:

2 oz. of vodka, classic

3 oz. of beer, ginger

1/2 lime, juice only, fresh

For garnishing – 1 lime wedge, fresh

Directions:

Add the vodka, then ginger beer & lime juice to a copper cocktail mug or a highball glass.

Fill the mug or glass using crushed ice.

Stir to combine well.

Use lime wedge for garnishing and serve.

Dirty Martini

Preparation time: 10 minutes

Servings: 2

Ingredients:

6 ounces vodka

1 ounce olive brine

1 dash dry vermouth

Ice cubes

4 stuffed green olives

Directions:

Shake vodka, olive brine, and dry vermouth.

Pour into a Collins glass.

Fill with ice cubes.

Garnish with green olives.

Caramel Spiced Tea

Preparation time: 5 minutes

Servings: 2

Ingredients:

1.5 ounces Smirnoff Kissed Caramel vodka

2 ounces unsweetened strong Chai tea

1 ounce half-and-half

0.5 ounces simple syrup

Ice cubes

Directions:

Shake vodka, strong Chai tea, half-and-half, and maple syrup.

Pour into a Collins glass.

Fill with ice cubes.

Pomegranate Berry Punch

Preparation time: 5 minutes

Servings: 2

Ingredients:

1.5 ounces Smirnoff sorbet light raspberry pomegranate vodka

1 ounce cranberry juice

2 ounces cocktail ginger ale

Ice cubes

1 lime wedge

Directions:

Shake Smirnoff vodka, cranberry juice, and cocktail ginger ale

Pour into a Collins glass.

Fill with ice cubes.

Garnish with lime wedges.

Honey Cider

Preparation time: 5 minutes

Servings: 2

Ingredients:

1.5 ounces Smirnoff wild honey vodka

2.5 ounces cider

2.5 ounces apple juice

Ice cubes

Directions:

Shake Smirnoff wild honey, cider, and apple juice.

Pour into a Collins glass.

Fill with ice cubes.

Black Cherry Bloom

Preparation time: 5 minutes

Servings: 2

Ingredients:

1 ounce blood orange Juice

¾ ounce lime juice

¾ ounce agave nectar

2 ounces black cherry vodka

3 sliced strawberry

4 mint leaves

1 pinch cayenne pepper

Ice cubed

For garnishing:

2 mint leaves

1 hulled strawberry

Directions:

Shake cherry vodka, blood orange juice, lime juice, and agave nectar.

Add vodka, strawberry, mint leaves, and cayenne pepper and shake with ice cubes.

Strain into a Collins glass and garnish with mint leaves and strawberry.

Red Tart

Preparation time: 5 minutes

Servings: 2

Ingredients:

1½ ounces red berry vodka

¾ ounce black raspberry liqueur

1 ounce amaretto

½ ounce lime juice

1 ounce lemon-lime soda

Ice cubes

Directions:

Shake vodka, black raspberry liqueur, amaretto, lime juice, and lemon-lime soda.

Pour into a Collins glass.

Fill with ice cubes.

Keto Liqueurs

Benedictine Blast Cocktail

Preparation time: 10 minutes

Servings: 3

Ingredients:

8 milliliters Benedictine D.O.M. liqueur

8 milliliters white crème de cacao liqueur

½ teaspoon mezcal

22 milliliters cold water

60 milliliters tequila

Directions:

Stir ingredients with ice and strain into chilled glass.

Cold Shower

Preparation time: 10 minutes

Servings: 2

Ingredients:

Creme de menthe (1 part, green)

Club soda (4 parts)

Directions:

1. In a highball glass add ice, club soda, and the creme de menthe then stir and enjoy.

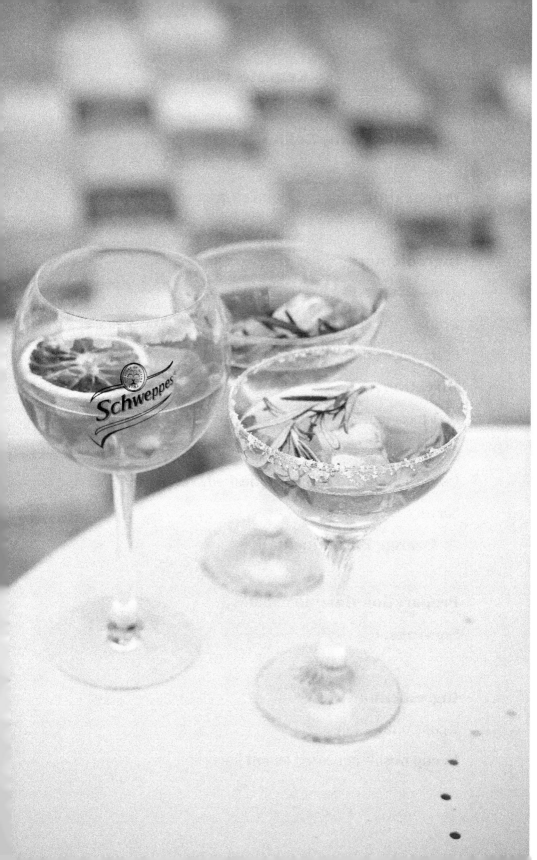

Keto Mocktails

No-Wine Baby Bellini

Preparation time: 4 minutes

Servings: 4

Ingredients:

2 ounces sparkling cider

2 ounces peach nectar

Peach slice for garnish (optional)

Directions:

Pour peach nectar into a champagne flute.

Add sparkling cider slowly.

Use peach slice to garnish, if desired.

Serve.

Orange Basil Mocktail

Preparation time: 10 minutes

Servings: 6

Ingredients:

2 cups orange juice

¼ cup freshly squeezed lemon juice

½ cup soda water

¼ cup water

2 tablespoons sugar

2-3 basil leaves

Ice cubes for serving

Orange slices for garnish

Directions:

In a pitcher, mix orange juice, lemon juice, soda water, water, sugar, and basil.

Spoon ice cubes into serving glasses and pour orange juice on top.

Garnish with orange slices and serve immediately.

Roy Rogers

Preparation time: 10 minutes

Servings: 4

Ingredients:

¼ ounce grenadine

8 ounces cola-flavored soda

1 maraschino strawberry for garnish

Directions:

Fill a tall glass with ice. Pour in grenadine.

Add cola and stir to combine.

Use maraschino strawberry for garnish and serve.

Sherbet Raspberry Mocktail

Preparation time: 10 minutes

Servings: 4

Ingredients:

2 cups Sprite

2 cups soda water

1 (12-ounce) can pink lemonade

½ cup pineapple wedges

½ cup raspberries

8 scoops of raspberry sherbet ice cream, frozen

Directions:

In a large glass bowl, mix the Sprite, soda water, lemonade, pineapple wedges, and raspberries.

Pour the drink into serving glasses and scoop one dollop of the ice cream onto each glass.

Enjoy immediately!

Strawberry Faux Daiquiri

Preparation time: 10 minutes

Servings: 4

Ingredients:

2 large strawberries

1 ½ pints orangeade

Crushed ice

1 small strawberry for garnish

Directions:

Hull strawberries.

Combine the crushed ice, strawberries, and orangeade in a blender.

Blend ingredients well. Pour in a glass.

Use strawberry for garnish.

Serve.

Tropical Fruits

Preparation time: 10 minutes

Servings: 4

Ingredients:

1 ¼ cup chopped strawberries

2 cups sparkling water

2 oranges juiced

Directions:

In a pitcher, add the strawberries and use a muddler to mash the fruits.

Pour in the sparkling water, orange juice, and cover the pitcher with plastic wrap.

Chill in the refrigerator for 2 hours.

Serve the drink in glasses.

Tuscan Fresco

Preparation time: 10 minutes

Servings: 1

Ingredients:

Ice made with filtered water

2 sprigs rosemary

1 ounce peach nectar

1 ounce white cranberry juice

½ ounce fresh orange juice

½ ounce store-bought simple syrup

1 ounce chilled club soda

Directions:

Add ice to the cocktail shaker till full.

Add a sprig of rosemary, along with the simple syrup, orange juice, cranberry juice, and peach nectar.

Shake to thoroughly combine. Strain into ice-filled glass.

Stir club soda. Use the remaining sprig of rosemary to garnish. Serve.

Mandarin Mojito Mocktail

Preparation time: 5 minutes

Servings: 3

Ingredients:

8 fluid oz of Sprite or 7UP

½ of a fluid oz of Mandarin Syrup

½ of a fluid oz of Mojito Mix

5 Mandarin orange segments

3-5 large mint leaves

1 lime

Mandarin orange segments as garnish

Directions:

Cut the lime into at least two wedges.

Place the 2 lime wedges, mint leaves & orange segments into your glass.

Muddle the ingredients.

Now place the rest of the ingredients into the glass.

Stir the drink mixture.

Add the desired amount of ice.

Use additional orange segments for garnish.

Virgin Bloody Mary with Shrimp

Preparation time: 5 minutes

Servings: 3

Ingredients:

22 oz of reduced-sodium V8

1 tsp of horseradish

1 tsp of Worcestershire sauce

1 Tbsp of lemon juice

10 dashes Tabasco

Freshly ground pepper, to taste

Ice cubes

4 cooked shrimp

Directions:

Combine the V8, Worcestershire sauce, horseradish, Tabasco, lemon juice & pepper into a glass jar.

Use the lid and shake.

Place ice into two tall glasses.

Evenly divide the drink mixture between the two glasses.

Use the two shrimp as garnish.

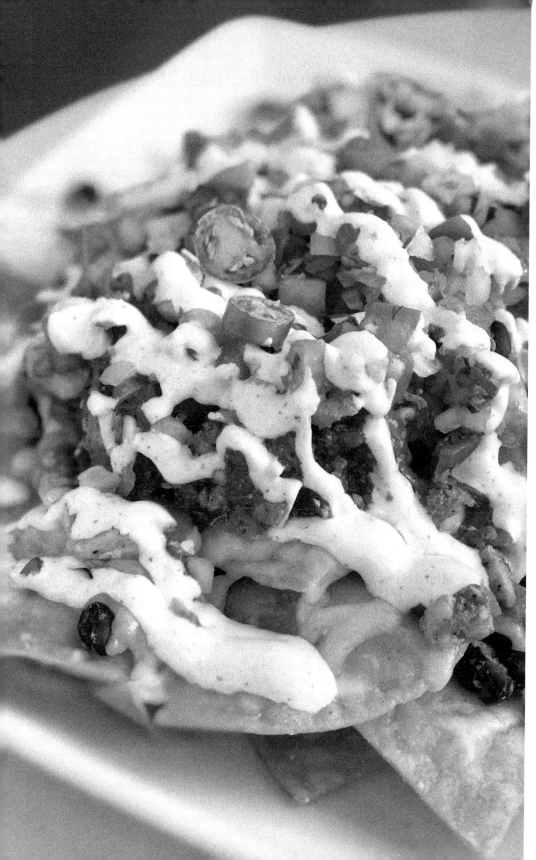

Keto Snacks for Happy Hour

Nutmeg Nougat

Preparation time: 30 minutes

Cooking Time: 60 minutes

Servings: 12

Ingredients:

1 Cup Heavy Cream

1 Cup Cashew Butter

1 Cup Coconut, Shredded

½ Teaspoon Nutmeg

1 Teaspoon Vanilla Extract, Pure

Stevia to Taste

Directions:

Melt your cashew butter using a double boiler, and then stir in your vanilla extract, dairy cream, nutmeg, and stevia. Make sure it's mixed well.

Remove from heat, allowing it to cool down before refrigerating it for half an hour.

Shape into balls, and coat with shredded coconut. Chill for at least two hours before serving.

Nutrition: calories 110, fat 10, fiber 1, carbs 3, protein 6

Sweet Almond Bites

Preparation time: 30 minutes

Cooking Time: 90 minutes

Servings: 12

Ingredients:

18 Ounces Butter, Grass-Fed

2 Ounces Heavy Cream

½ Cup Stevia

2/3 Cup Cocoa Powder

1 Teaspoon Vanilla Extract, Pure

4 Tablespoons Almond Butter

Directions:

Use a double boiler to melt your butter before adding in all of your remaining ingredients.

Place the mixture into molds, freezing for two hours before serving.

Lemon Fat Bombs

Preparation time: 10 minutes

Cooking Time: 50 minutes

Servings: 4

Ingredients:

1 cup of shredded coconut (dry)

1/4 cup of coconut oil

3 tbsps. of erythritol sweetener (powdered)

1 tbsps. of lemon zest

1 pinch of salt

Directions:

Add the coconut to a high-power blender. Blend until creamy for fifteen minutes. Add sweetener, coconut oil, salt, and lemon zest. Blend for two minutes. Fill small muffin cups with the coconut mixture. Chill in the refrigerator for thirty minutes.

Nutrition: calories 200, fat 8, fiber 4, carbs 8, protein 3

Thousand Island Salad Dressing

Preparation time: 5 minutes

Cooking Time: 5 minutes

Servings: 8 servings

Ingredients:

2 Tbsp. olive oil

¼ c frozen spinach, thawed.

2 T dried parsley

1 T dried dill

1 t onion powder

½ t salt

¼ t black pepper

1 c full-fat mayonnaise

¼ c full-fat sour cream

Directions:

Combine all ingredients in a small mixing bowl.

Nutrition: calories 383, fat 14, fiber 4, carbs 3, protein 8

Keto Salad Niçoise

Preparation time: 5 minutes

Cooking Time: 5 minutes

Servings: 4

Ingredients:

2 eggs

2 oz. celery root

4 oz. green beans

2 tablespoons olive oil

2 garlic cloves

4 oz. romaine lettuce

2 oz. cherry tomatoes

¼ red onion

1 can tuna

2 oz. olives

Dressing

2 tablespoons capers

¼ oz. anchovies

½ cup olive oil

½ cup mayonnaise

¼ lemon

1 tablespoon parsley

Directions:

In a bowl sauté peppers in coconut oil. In a bowl add all ingredients and mix well. Serve with dressing

Nutrition: calories 110, fat 10, fiber 1, carbs 3, protein 6

Greek Salad

Preparation time: 5 minutes

Cooking Time: 5 minutes

Servings: 4

Ingredients:

2 ripe tomatoes

¼ cucumber

¼ red onion

¼ green bell pepper

6 oz. feta cheese

8 black Greek olives

5 tablespoons olive oil

¼ tablespoon red wine vinegar

2 tsp oregano

Directions:

In a bowl add all ingredients and mix well. Serve with dressing

Nutrition: calories 383, fat 14, fiber 4, carbs 3, protein 8

Conclusion

Here we come to the end of our journey with keto cocktails. In addition to being really delicious, these cocktails will also help you lose weight and counteract some diseases. Obviously remember to drink enough water. Any ketogenic plan can cause mild or severe dehydration, which could lead to other health complications. Water also helps you lose weight, which is all the more reason to hydrate yourself throughout the day. Have the ingredients ready to make a quick drink on the go. This will help you stay on track and stick to your goals.

CPSIA information can be obtained
at www.ICGtesting.com
Printed in the USA
BVHW041349250621
610376BV00008B/1649